Mediterranean Definitive Cookbook

The Ultimate Collection of Delicious Mediterranean Recipes

Valerie Reynolds

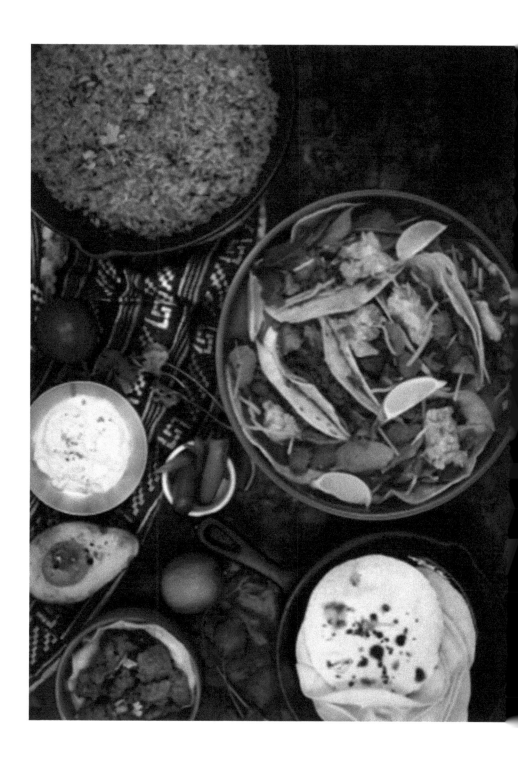

By reading this document, the reader agrees that under no circumstances is the author responsible for any losses, direct or indirect, which are incurred as a result of the use of information contained within this document, including, but not limited to, — errors, omissions, or inaccuracies.

Table of Contents

Spinach and cheddar quiche

Enjoy this absolutely meat free pie recipe possible to serve as an appetizer or main dish as well. It is fully stuffed with veggies, cream mixture, and an egg topped with cheese achieve the sweetness that you are seeking for in 50 minutes.

Ingredients

2 eggs

1½ cup of all-purpose flour

1 leek

½ stick of unsalted butter

1 small egg

¼ teaspoon of black pepper

3 tablespoons of cold water

¾ cup of milk

2 teaspoons of vegetable oil

A pinch of salt

2 cups pf frozen spinach

½ teaspoon of salt

½ cup of half and half

1 small red onion

2 ounces of grated cheese

Directions

Start with the crust, therefore, Place flour, chilled diced butter, and salt in a food processor.

Process until crumb-like texture.

Add the egg and cold water continue to process until the dough pulls together.

Remove out and wrap in a cling-film

Refrigerate for 20 – 30 minutes.

As it refrigerates, dice the onion.

Cut the leek in half length-wise. Further cut each half again, chop.

Pour oil in a skillet, add the onion together with the leek. Sauté for 5 minutes on medium temperature.

Add the frozen spinach continue to Sauté for more 5 minutes.

Turn off the heat.

Add seasoning stir frequently.

In a medium sized bowl, whisk the eggs, milk, and half and half until fully combined.

Grate the cheese.

Take out the pastry, divide into 2 pieces. Neatly roll out each of them ensure to make then larger than the pan bottom due to the need to cover them.

Make sure to line the pans with baking parchment and grease the sides with butter.

Place the crust pastry in.

With your hands, press the pastry down and to the sides.

With the back of your knife cut off the excess pastry.

Divide the filling into two equal halves and spread onto each pastry.

Pour the egg mixture over, top with cheese.

Proceed to bake in a preheated oven at 180° for 25 minutes.

Serve and enjoy.

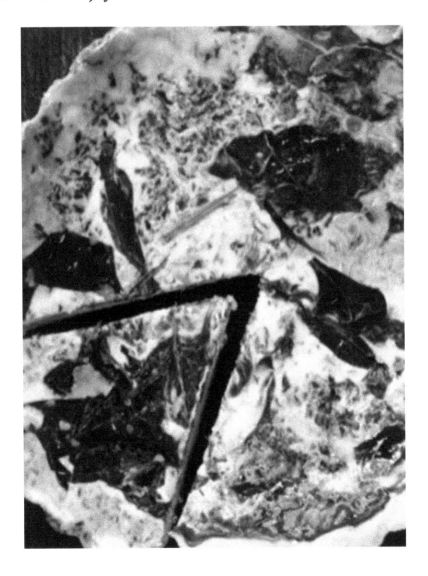

Artichoke tart

Cooked with spring onions and prosciutto, this artichoke tart is perfect for anyone. It utilizes range of ingredients and flavors topped with juicy tomatoes and roasted with roasted peppers.

Ingredients

2 tablespoon of roasted red pepper pesto

1 teaspoon of rosemary , optional

6 slices of prosciutto

½ cup of cheddar cheese (50g)

8 cherry tomatoes

1 puff pastry sheet

½ cup of green olives

2 spring onions

2 chili peppers

1 cup of artichoke hearts

Directions

Preheat your oven ready to 200°.

Roll out the pastry and cut in half.

Place both puff pastry sheets onto a baking tray lined with parchment paper.

Endeavor to ensure there is space in between the sheets.

Using a pizza cutter carefully cut out a rectangle ½ inch on both pastries from the edges.

Spread pesto over the pastry sheets.

Sprinkle cheese over and top each with the rest of the remaining ingredients.

Bake in the preheated oven for 12 minutes.

Serve and enjoy.

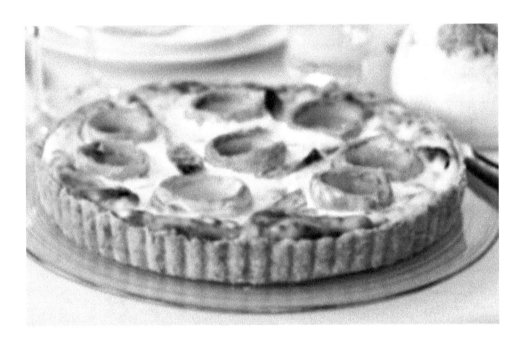

Vegetarian fresh spring rolls with peanut sauce

Using peanut butter as a dipping option for the vegetable spring rolls makes this recipe quite unique. The raw veggies are boosted by the salty feta cheese with its great aromatic refreshing healthy flavor.

Ingredients

Feta cheese

2 medium carrots

1 teaspoon of soy sauce

1 large yellow/red bell pepper

2 cups of baby kale leaves

¼ head of purple cabbage

2 tablespoons of water

2 medium avocados

4 tablespoons of peanut butter

1 small lemon

2 tablespoons of honey

6 rice paper sheets

Directions

Prepare the veggies by cutting the pepper and carrots into matchsticks.

Slice avocados and cabbage as thinly.

Remove any hard stems from baby kale leaves.

In a large frying pan, place warm water in to soak the rice paper until soft in about 20 seconds or more. Remove when the rice paper has completely softened when felt.

Place the soften paper onto a clean work top and add the fillings beginning at the bottom ⅓ of the paper.

Crumble some Feta cheese over it, add some carrots, peppers, and cabbage.

Roll the fillings in the paper as if you are wrapping. Nevertheless, only roll to close the first batch.

Add more fillings mainly the avocado and the kale, once you have finished rolling.

Hold the fillings with your hands as you roll the roll away while tucking the fillings in.

Close both edges by folding the rice paper in and complete the rolling.

Keep pressing the roll to ensure the fillings are not loose.

Combine all the ingredients until smooth, for the peanut butter after softening in a microwave.

Serve immediately and enjoy.

Cheese tortellini pasta with broccoli and bacon

Just reserve 20 minutes to complete making this cheese tortellini pasta with broccoli and bacon using only 5 ingredients.

Ingredients

16 ounces of fresh cheese tortellini
1 cup of single cream
2 cups of bacon slices (200 grams)
2 cups of cheddar cheese or similar, grated
2 cups of broccoli florets

Directions

Boil a large pot of water.
Throw in tortellini and broccoli.
Cook until ready in 5 minutes or according to the package instruction of the tortellini.
Fry the bacon.
Pour in cream as you stir.
Reduce the heat as the sauce thickens, stir in grated cheese.
Turn off the source of heat.
Drain excess water in the tortellini and broccoli.
Pour the cheesy bacon sauce over and mix
Serve warm and enjoy with cheese though optional.

Simple campfire stew

If you have a crowd to feed do not look further. Here is the right recipe to handle a crowd.

Ingredients

3 tablespoon of Salt

1.1 lb. of Boston Butt or Pork Shoulder

3 lb. of Potatoes

4.5 lb. of Beef Round Steak

3 tablespoon of Dried Marjoram

11 cups of Water

Dried of Fresh Chili Pepper, optional

4 Garlic Cloves

1 can of Beer

½ cup of Lard

4 tablespoon of Caraway Seeds

1½ lb. of Onion

2½ tablespoon of Sweet Paprika

1 tablespoon of Tomato Paste

Directions

In large pot, melt the lard.

Add diced onion and sauté for 5 minutes.

Add the meats diced into small pieces.

Let them brown as you stir occasionally.

Add sweet paprika, toss to mix well, let cook for 1 minute.

Add 4 cups water, caraway seeds, salt, ½ of diced potatoes, and 1 can of beer.

Cover with lid tightly let cook as you keep checking once in a time.

Keep checking the amount of water, add accordingly, continue to simmer for 1 hour and 30 minutes then add the rest of the potatoes, add water accordingly.

Cook until the meat is ready.

Add the tomato paste, marjoram, minced garlic, and dried whole chili, when the meat is about to get ready to flavor it.

Taste and season accordingly.

Serve when warm with slices of bread.

Enjoy.

Spicy spaghetti aglio olio and pepperoncino

Ingredients

Chili

1 cup of parmesan cheese, grated

5 - 6 tablespoon of extra virgin olive oil

1 pounds Spaghetti

2 cups of fresh flat leaf parsley, chopped

10 - 12 cloves Garlic

Salt

Directions

Start off with boiling water for spaghetti.

When the water is boiling, add salt and spaghetti cook as instructed on the package by the manufacturer

As the spaghetti is boiling, rinse parsley and chili.

Chop all of them finely.

Peel and thinly chop garlic.

Grate Parmesan.

When the spaghetti is about to get ready, heat oil in a frying pan.

Add garlic, sauté for 2 minutes on low temperature while stirring infrequently.

place in the parsley together with the chili and some tablespoons of pasta water allow it cook for 2 minutes.

Drain spaghetti of excess water and pour the sauce over it.

Sprinkle with Parmesan

Serve and enjoy.

Cauliflower bake with blue cheese and prosciutto

This recipe turns the ordinary veggie to something remarkably delicious using as an appetizer with blue cheese.

Ingredients

3 carrots

1 egg

4 tablespoon of olive oil

1 small onion, diced

4 prosciutto

1 pounds of cauliflower

2 tablespoons of bread crumbs

¼ cup of fresh flat leaf parsley, finely chopped

Salt and pepper

¼ cup of blue cheese

Instruction

Wash the carrots well, peel and grate.

Secondly, wash the cauliflower, remove any green parts. Chop into smaller pieces

Place in food processor, process until crumb like texture forms.

In a large bowl, blend processed cauliflower, carrots, diced onion, seasoning, breadcrumbs and the egg.

In a frying pan, heat the oil and sauté the cauliflower mixture for 5 minutes, keep stirring occasionally.

Stir in the fresh parsley.

Line a square sandwich pan with baking parchment paper.

Fill the bottom with half of the cauliflower mixture.

Push it down with the back of a spoon.

Add prosciutto torn into smaller pieces together with the crumbled cheese.

Cover tightly with the rest of the cauliflower mixture, again push it down to the bottom.

Now bake in already heated oven for 15 minutes.

Serve and enjoy as an appetizer or side dish.

Spinach crepes with pan-roasted vegetables

Ginger with its strong aromatic flavor is used for topping in this recipe with mushrooms, pepper, tomatoes and onions in 30 minutes of total preparation time. It is perfect for diner, lunch and even breakfast.

Ingredients
1 cup of milk
1 cup of plain flour
1 teaspoon pink Himalayan salt
½ teaspoon of pink Himalayan salt
1 thumb-size piece of fresh ginger, grated
1 cup of grated cheese of your choice
3 tablespoons of butter
2 cups of chopped mushrooms
1 yellow bell pepper
4 cups of fresh spinach
1 medium onion
2 cups of cherry tomatoes
2 cups of chopped flat leaf parsley
1 cup of grated cheese of your choice
1 tablespoon dried oregano
1 large egg
3 garlic cloves

Sunflower oil for frying

Directions

In a food processor, blend the spinach together with the milk until smooth.

Pour the mixture in a bowl.

Add flour, egg, salt, and grated ginger, then whisk till well combined.

Heat up the frying pan.

Add a little oil and place in the batter.

Spread around evenly

Once set, turn it over and cook for 1 minute.

Melt the butter in a frying pan.

Add sliced mushrooms, onion, and pepper.

Roast for 10 minutes then add the cherry tomatoes together with garlic.

Continue to roast for more 2 – 3 minutes.

Switch off the heat.

Stir in the parsley.

Fill pancakes with vegetable mixture.

Sprinkle with grated cheese.

Serve when warm and enjoy.

Baked curry chicken wings with mango chutney

The mango chutney is used to perfectly marinate the chicken wings when they have become very tender and then baked for dinner, lunch or breakfast.

Ingredients

⅔ cup of mango chutney

2.5 pounds of chicken wings

4 tablespoons of curry powder

2 tablespoon of oyster sauce

2 tablespoons of Worcestershire sauce

Teaspoons of pink Himalayan salt

Instruction

Place chicken wings in a bowl.

Season with salt and curry powder.

Mix well to ensure even coating.

In a separate bowl combine the Worcestershire sauce, mango chutney, and oyster sauce.

Pour gently over wings, mix until each piece is well coated in the sauce.

Cover the bowl with a close zip-lock bag and refrigerate for not less than 30 minutes.

After it is marinated, put the wings onto a baking tray lined with baking paperwith enough space between them.

Spoon the marinade over the wings.

Bake in a preheated oven at 200° for 25 minutes.

Serve and enjoy with a dip of your liking.

10-minute bake bean pasta sauce

Ingredients

A handful of fresh flat leaf parsley

1 can of tomato pasta

1 can of baked beans in tomato sauce

3.5 oz. of cheddar cheese

3 garlic cloves

4.5 oz. of chorizo

Instruction

Begin by chop chorizo into smaller pieces.

Place in a frying pan do not add all oil because it has its own fat that will melt.

Peel and slice garlic cloves put to the chorizo.

Cook for 5 minutes as you stir occasionally.

Add the tomato pasta together with the baked beans.

Lower the heat let simmer for 5 minutes.

Put in the finely chopped parsley when it is about to get ready.

Turn off the heat and stir in cheese

Serve immediately with pasta.

Enjoy.

Sweet chili pesto burger sliders

This recipe combines sweet chili sauce, pesto, tomatoes, salad leaves and pesto burgers among other ingredients for a tasty breakfast to boost your healthy in 30 minutes' periods.

Ingredients

Mixed salad leaves or lamb lettuce

¼ teaspoon of pink Himalayan salt

1 lb. of minced beef (440g)

¼ teaspoon of black pepper

9 mini burger buns

2 tomatoes

3 tablespoons of green pesto

2 tablespoons of pesto

Sweet chili sauce to your taste

1 egg

Directions

In a bowl, mix pepper, salt, pesto, minced beef, and eggs. Form into patties by rolling the mixture into a bowl, after which you flatten them, make less than 11 patties.

Place each patty on a baking tray lined with baking paper.

Move them to the oven heated to 190° and bake for 20 minutes.

Cut each bun in half.

Spread over with sweet chili sauce.

Add lamb lettuce together with tomato slice and a teaspoon of pesto.

Followed by burger patty and more lettuce.

Cover with bun.

Pierce with burger skewer.

Serve and enjoy.

Whole wheat crispy popcorn chicken wrap

Whole wheat as a food is a healthy and nutritious with high fiber and carbohydrate content to boost a person's energy. In this recipe, it is used to coat the chicken wrapped with veggies.

Ingredients

¼ cabbage

1 tomato

1 green bell pepper

1 romaine lettuce

6 whole wheat tortillas

7 ounces of popcorn chicken

Directions

Begin by rinsing the veggies under running water.

Thinly slice cabbage and so the romaine lettuce.

Dice tomatoes and peppers.

Place everything in a mixing bowl mix to combine.

Next, deep-fry the homemade popcorn chicken as per the manufacturer Directions.

Place tortilla onto a plate and spread the salad across the middle.

Add popcorn chicken and roll the tortilla over the filling to coat.

Cut in half and wrap in a piece of baking parchment. Serve immediately and enjoy.

Nourishing Buddha bowl

Nourishing as the name suggests, this recipe is rich in nutrient though light meal. It only takes 25 minutes to get ready making it a quick meal which can also be prepared ahead.

Ingredients

1 baby romaine lettuce

6 tablespoons of natural yogurt or sour cream

1.7 ounces of buckwheat

2 tablespoons of unsalted butter

2 tablespoons of ketchup

2 avocados (medium)

2 spring onions (scallions)

2 carrots

Drizzle of lemon juice

1 teaspoon of sweet paprika

3 ounces of chickpea cooked

Drizzle of extra virgin olive oil

½-1 teaspoon of Himalayan salt to taste

Directions

Start by cooking the buckwheat as instructed by the manufacturer.

When ready, Season the water with ½ teaspoon salt.

As it cooks, rinse all the vegetables.

Peel and slice carrots.

Cut the spring onions and lettuce.

Cut avocado in half, remove the seed then scoop out using a spoon.

Cut it into strips

Melt the butter in a pan.

Add in drained chickpea let roast for 3 minutes.

Add sweet paprika toss around until all the chickpeas are coated evenly.

Continue to roast for more 2 minutes.

Turn off the heat.

Taste and season accordingly.

Arrange all the ingredients in a bowl, serve warm with a lemon wedge and extra virgin olive oil.

Enjoy.

Mini vegetarian puff pastry pizzas

The mini vegetarian puff pastry pizza will be ready in not more than 10 minutes topped with fresh vegetables and arugula as well as cheese.

Ingredients

A handful of fresh arugula

1 batch homemade pizza sauce

6 cherry tomatoes, thinly sliced

½ small onion, thinly sliced

1 chili pepper, thinly sliced

6 olives, thinly sliced

1 puff pastry sheet

6 goat cheese, thin slices (optional)

1 small zucchini, sliced

1 ounce blue cheese

Directions

Preheat your oven to 200°.

As the oven heats, roll out the puff pastry sheet so thin. Using a 4-inch round cookie cutter, cut out many circles. Place them onto a baking tray lined with baking parchment.

Use an inch smaller cutter to make smaller circles inside the pastry, make sure not to cut through.

Top the pastry circles with a teaspoon of pizza sauce each piece, cherry tomatoes, some slices of zucchini, olives, little onion, and goat cheese and or blue cheese. Sprinkle with chili pepper

Repeat this process and then bake at 200° for 10 – 15 minutes.

Top with arugula though optional but it is good.

Serve and enjoy.

Savory crepes with chia seeds and garlic

Savory crepes can be made nicely with minced meat with some canned tomatoes and variety of vegetables. Milk, rye and garlic with chia seeds elevate this recipe to the next level.

Ingredients

¼ tsp salt

½ cup rye flour

2 cups milk

1 tablespoon of dried oregano

1 tablespoon of chia seeds

3 cloves garlic

½ cup plain flour

1 medium egg

Directions

In a bowl, combine all the ingredients mix until you get a smooth batter

Heat a frying pan over a moderate temperature.

Add some oil in the pan.

Pour in the batter, then spread evenly by tilting the pan to all directions

Place in the pancakes until a visible golden brown color underneath.

Cook for more 1 – 2 minutes.

Move all to a plate when ready.

Serve and enjoy.

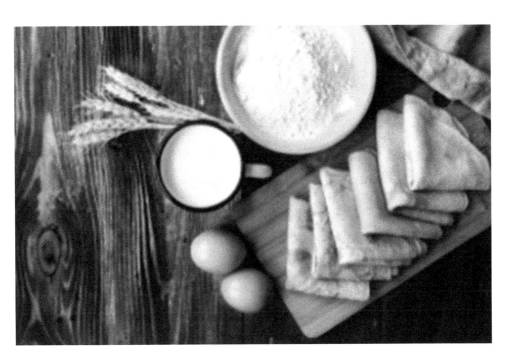

Panko salmon with snap peas

Ingredients

Prepared with Dijon mustard, this simple fresh tarragon kicks in with a sweet anise-y flavor. The salmon seared crusted side down is much easier to flip when golden and crispy. Snap peas are sweeter when crisp tender as this recipe just makes it.

Ingredients

½ tablespoon of Dijon mustard

½ teaspoon of canola mayonnaise

½ teaspoon of black pepper divided

¾ teaspoon of kosher salt

4 skinless of salmon fillets

1 tablespoon of chopped fresh tarragon

½ cup of whole wheat panko

2 teaspoons of grated lemon rind

2 tablespoon of olive oil

1/3 cup of thinly sliced shallots

2 teaspoon of fresh lemon juice

2 cups of sugar snap peas, trimmed

Directions

Start by combining mayonnaise, ½ teaspoon of salt, mustard, and ¼ teaspoon of pepper in a shallow bowl. Spoon mustard mixture evenly over fillets.

Combine panko with 1 teaspoon of tarragon, and 1 teaspoon of the lemon rind in a bowl.

Sprinkle panko mixture over fillets ensure to press down to combine.

Heat 1 tablespoon of oil in a large skillet over medium temperature.

Add panko side down, fillets, to the heated pan let cook for 3 – 4 minutes

Turnover, continue to cook for more 3 – 4 minutes.

Remove from heat source and keep warm

Increase heat to high.

Add remaining 1 tablespoon of oil to pan.

Add snap peas and shallots let cook for 3 minutes as you keep stirring occasionally.

Add remaining ¼ teaspoon of salt, 1 teaspoon of lemon rind, ¼ teaspoon of pepper, ½ teaspoons of tarragon, and juice to pan

Let cook for 2 minutes until crisp-tender.

Serve with fillets.

Enjoy.

Arugula and cremini quiche with gluten-free almond meal crust

This is a gourmet simple recipe for any meal whether lunch, dinner or breakfast. It combines gluten-free thyme, almond meal crust, arugula and cremini mushrooms along with goat cheese to give a tasty feel in the taste buds.

Ingredients

5 ounces of goat cheese, crumbled

3 garlic cloves, pressed or minced

3 cups of baby arugula, roughly chopped

2 cups of packed almond meal or almond flour

⅓ cup of milk

¼ teaspoon of red pepper flakes

¼ teaspoon of freshly ground pepper

1 tablespoon of and 1 teaspoon water

1 ½ cups of cleaned and sliced Cremini mushrooms

⅓ cup of olive oil

1 teaspoon of salt

Drizzle olive oil

6 large eggs

1 tablespoon of minced fresh thyme or 1 teaspoon dried thyme

Directions

Preheat oven to 400°F.

Oil a cast iron skillet with olive oil.

In a mixing bowl, stir together the garlic, thyme, almond meal, salt and pepper.

Pour in the olive oil and water, stir to combine them mixture.

Press the dough into your prepared skillet evenly across the bottom at least 1 ¼ inch up the sides.

Bake until the crust is lightly golden and firm to the touch in 15 – 20 minutes.

In a large oven at high temperature, warm enough olive oil to lightly coat the pan.

Cook the mushrooms with a dash of salt, stir often till it becomes tender.

Toss in the arugula and let it wilt, keep stirring for 3o seconds.

Move the mixture to a plate, let cool.

In another mixing bowl, whisk together the milk, eggs, salt and red pepper.

Gently stir in the goat cheese together with the slightly cooled mushroom and arugula mixture.

After baking the crust, pour in the egg mixture, let bake for 30 minutes.

Allow the quiche to cool for 5 or 10 minutes

Slice with a sharp knife.

Serve immediately and enjoy.

Huevos rancheros with avocado salsa Verde

Black beans together with fresh creamy avocado make this delicious rancheros recipe. It is healthy and tasty for a great dinner. Meatless but packed with veggies, this makes a great Mediterranean Sea diet.

Ingredients

½ lime, halved

1 tablespoon of olive oil

½ teaspoon of chili powder

¼ teaspoon of cayenne pepper

1 lime, halved

½ cup of feta, crumbled

½ jalapeño, seeds, membranes removed, finely chopped

Salt and pepper

2 cans pf black black beans, rinsed and drained

1 cup of mild salsa Verde

4 or more eggs

1 ripe avocado, pitted and sliced

½ medium red onion, chopped

1 medium jalapeño, deseeded and roughly chopped

4 radishes, sliced into thin pieces

Hot sauce

1 garlic clove, chopped

4 or more corn tortillas

Big handful of cilantro

Small handful cilantro, chopped

½ teaspoon of cumin powder

Directions

Begin by cook the beans.

Heat a drizzle of olive oil in a medium saucepan that has a lid over medium heat.

After the oil is warmed, add the onion let sauté for some minutes ensure to stir frequently till onions become translucent.

Add the chili cumin, powder, and cayenne blend.

Add the beans in ¼ cup of water stir to combine.

Cover the pan, reduce heat, let the beans cook by simmering for 10 minutes.

Remove from heat, mash some of the beans with the back of a big spoon.

Keep the pan until the meal is ready to serve.

Next, make the avocado salsa Verde by using a food processor.

In the food processor, combine the salsa Verde, cilantro, avocado, garlic clove, ½ of the jalapeño, and the juice of ½ lime.

Purée the salsa until it is super creamy.

Transfer the salsa Verde to a small saucepan and gently warm it over medium-low temperature as you stir frequently.

Cover the salsa and keep until you are ready to serve

Prepare the eggs and top with a light sprinkle of salt and pepper.

Warm the tortillas over low temperature gas.

Assemble the huevos rancheros by placing nn each plate, top tortilla with black beans, avocado sauce and egg.

Garnish with cilantro, chopped radishes, crumbled feta, and jalapeño.

Serve and enjoy with a bottle of hot sauce on the side.

Pumpkin pecan scones with maple glaze

Topped with a delightful maple glaze, this whole wheat pumpkin pecan makes a perfect healthy meal for your entire family in 30 minutes.

Ingredients

¾ cup of pumpkin puree

¼ cup of good maple syrup

½ teaspoon of vanilla extract

2 cups of white whole wheat flour

½ teaspoon of ginger

½ teaspoon of salt

1 cup of raw pecans

⅓ cup of solid coconut oil

¼ cup of milk of choice

1 teaspoon of cinnamon

¼ teaspoon of cloves or allspices

1 cup of powdered sugar

1 tablespoon of baking powder

¼ teaspoon of nutmeg

⅛ teaspoon of fine grain sea salt

¼ cup of brown sugar, packed

1 tablespoon of melted coconut oil or butter

½ teaspoon of vanilla

Directions

Preheat your oven to 425°F.

Place the nuts in a single layer on a rimmed baking sheet lined with parchment paper.

Toast the nuts in the oven for 3 minutes until fragrant.

Chop the nuts into fine pieces.

Combine the¾ of the chopped nuts, baking powder, flour, spices, sugar, and salt in a bowl then whisk at once.

Using a pastry cutter, cut the coconut oil into the dry ingredients.

Stir in pumpkin puree together with the milk and vanilla extract.

Mixing until you have thoroughly incorporated the wet and dry ingredients.

Form dough into a circle about an inch deep around.

Cut the circle into 8 even slices.

Separate slices and place on the baking sheet covered with parchment paper.

Bake for 15 – 17 minutes.

As the scones bake, whisk together the glaze ingredients in a small bowl until it forms a visible smooth and creamy.

Drizzle generously over the scones

While the glaze is wet, sprinkle it with the remaining chopped nuts.

Serve and enjoy.

Tex-Mex omelet with roasted cherry tomato salsa

The omelet is fully stuffed with black beans, chips topped with roasted cherry tomato salsa. It is perfect for breakfast, dinner and lunch in only 40 minutes.

Ingredients

⅓ cup of loosely packed cilantro, chopped

2 cloves garlic, minced

1 small lime, juiced

Sliced avocado

⅛ teaspoon of sea salt

2 tablespoons of milk or water

Hot sauce

Pinch of sea salt

Pinch of black pepper

Sour cream

Hot sauce

1 pint of cherry tomatoes

1 jalapeño, deseeded and membranes removed chopped

1 scant tablespoon butter

⅓ cup Jack cheese or other melty cheese

½ small white onion, chopped

3 tablespoons black beans

2 eggs

½ teaspoon of olive oil

handful blue corn chips or tortilla chips, broken into small pieces

Directions

start by making the salsa by preheating the oven to 400°F.

Line a small, rimmed baking pan with parchment paper for easy cleaning.

Toss the cherry tomatoes and ½ teaspoon of olive oil together with a Sprinkle of sea salt on the baking pan.

Roast for 15 – 20 minutes to the extent the tomatoes are juicy and collapsing easily.

In another separate bowl, mix together the cilantro, chopped onion, jalapeño, lime juice or vinegar, garlic, and sea salt.

Use a serrated knife to chop the tomatoes once they have cooled off.

Pull off the tomato skins for a smoother salsa.

Mix the tomatoes into the mixture.

Taste and season accordingly.

Secondly, it is time to make the omelet.

In a bowl, whisk together the milk or water, eggs, black pepper, sea salt, and dashes of hot sauce.

Heat a well-seasoned cast iron skillet over medium-low heat.

Add a drop of water sizzles on contact when the skillet is hot.

Toss in the pat of butter tilt to all sides to coat.

Pour in the egg mixture and let it set for briefly.

Using a spatula, scoot the eggs toward the middle of the pan, make sure to tilt the pan so runny eggs take their place.

Repeat this process until there is hardly any runny eggs to scoot.

Using your spatula again, release the underside of the omelet from the pan.

Keep tilting the pan to prevent the omelet form sticking on the pan.

Let it set briefly, then scoop it off the pan to a plate

Immediately top ½ of the warm omelet with a sprinkle of cheese.

Then with smashed tortilla chips, black beans, and more cheese.

Gently fold the other half on top.

Spoon a generous amount of salsa over the middle of the omelet.

Serve immediately and enjoy.

Banana trail mix

Coconut, oats, naturally sweetened honey give this recipe an elevated taste. Feel free to top this banana trail mix bread with nuts, dry fruits and serve with Greek yogurt to pull out all the sweetness to excite your taste buds.

Ingredients

¼ cup of honey

1 large egg

¾ cup of whole wheat pastry flour

¼ cup of chopped dark chocolate

½ cup of oats

1 ½ teaspoons of baking powder

½ cup of virgin coconut oil, melted

1 tablespoon of turbinado sugar

1 teaspoon of vanilla extract

½ cup of pecans, toasted and chopped

½ teaspoon of cinnamon

¾ cup of unsweetened shredded coconut, divided

⅓ cup of chopped candied ginger

⅓ cup of chopped dried cherries or cranberries

¼ teaspoon of table salt

1 cup of mashed ripe banana

Directions

Expressly begin by preheating your oven to 375°F.

Grease your loaf pan.

In a medium sized bowl, whisk the flour together with, baking powder, oats, salt and cinnamon.

Stir in ½ cup of shredded coconut, immediately mix in the pecans, chopped ginger, dried fruit, and dark chocolate.

In a separate bowl, also whisk the coconut oil together with the mashed banana, egg, honey, and vanilla.

Mix the wet ingredients together with the dry ingredients keep stirring until properly combined.

Place the batter into the loaf pan.

Sprinkle with the remaining ¼ cup of coconut.

Then top with a light sprinkle of turbinado (raw) sugar.

Bake until the toothpick inserted into the center comes out clean in 50 minutes.

Allow the bread cool in the pan, then you can slice.

Serve and enjoy.

Maple cinnamon applesauce

An apple a say keeps the doctor far away!!! In 20 minutes you will be able to keep the doctor as far away as possible. Serve it with oat meal or pancakes for a nutritious healthy breakfast.

Ingredients

1 tablespoon of ground cinnamon

¼ cup of and 2 tablespoons real maple syrup

Dash of sea salt

3 Gala apples

1 tablespoon of fresh lemon juice

3 Granny Smith or pippin apples

Directions

Of course you must start by peeling, core and chopping the apples into chunks.

In a heavy Dutch oven heated to a medium temperature, combine the apple chunks, together with the cinnamon, maple syrup, and lemon juice.

Cover tightly and let simmer for 12 minutes to soften the apples slightly.

Uncover the pot, continue cooking as you stir occasionally to break up the larger chunks in 5 – 10 minutes or accordingly.

Remove from heat source, you can add more maple syrup, cinnamon or lemon juice to suit your taste. Serve warm or chilled.

Enjoy.

Keep leftover in the fridge after is has cooled to room temperature.

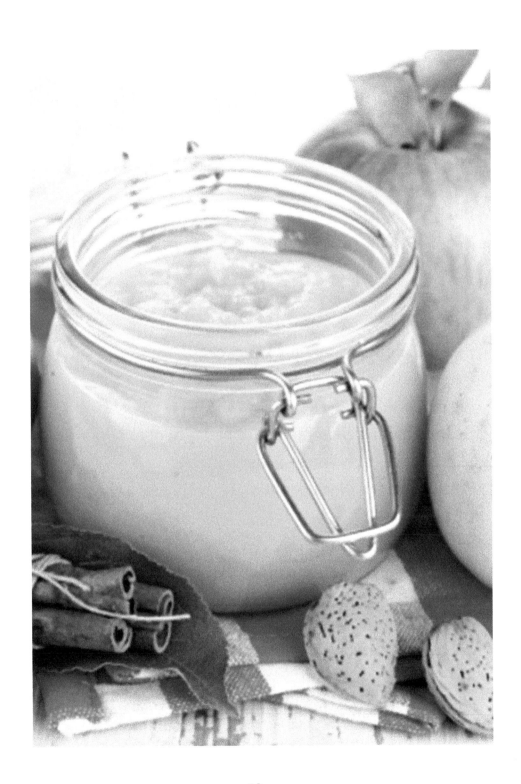

Baked asparagus frittata

This is one of a kind beautiful baked asparagus frittata recipe, very easy to make yet can make 6 larger servings.

Ingredients

Pinch of sea salt

1 ½ teaspoons of Dijon mustard

⅓ cup of milk

½ cup of crumbled goat cheese

6 large eggs

Handful of thin asparagus

Drizzle olive oil

Big pinch salt

Heaping tablespoon finely chopped shallot

Big squeeze fresh lemon juice

Freshly ground black pepper

Directions

Preheat oven to 400°F.

Secondly, line a baking pan with two strips of parchment paper trimmed to fit.

In a medium sized bowl, scramble the eggs together with the shallot, milk, mustard, goat cheese, and salt.

Pour the egg mixture into the prepared baking pan.

Carefully slide it onto the middle rack of the oven.

Bake for 10 minutes.

As the eggs are baking, rinse the asparagus and pat dry.

Trim off the tough ends of the asparagus.

Toss the asparagus with a big squeeze of lemon juice, salt, a drizzle of olive oil, and pepper.

Keep aside for later.

In 10 minutes, remove the egg dish from the oven.

Place the asparagus, one by one, on top.

Return back the rack to the oven for 15 minutes.

Let the frittata rest for a few minutes.

Next, slide a knife around the edges of the pan

Using both your hands, lift the frittata out and put onto a flat surface.

With a sharp knife slice it in three columns, in between the strips of asparagus.

Gently slice down the middle, through the asparagus.

Serve warm or at room temperature.

Enjoy.

Buckwheat and spelt crepes

Using a food processor these crepes are easier to whip, or even by hand and they really do not take long to get ready. They are blessed with a nutty flavor and amazing with savory eggs, butter and some fruity fillings. In 22 minutes your buckwheat and spelt crepes will be ready for breakfast, dinner and or desert depending on how you like it.

Ingredients

¾ cup of plus 2 tablespoons milk

1 tablespoon of unsalted butter, melted

¼ cup of buckwheat flour

½ cup of whole spelt flour

2 large eggs

¼ teaspoon of salt

2 teaspoons of sugar

Directions

In a food processor, combine the sugar, flours, and salt. Pulse it briefly to combine.

Add the milk to the content together with the eggs and melted butter.

Pour the liquid ingredients into the food processor blend till the mixture is uniform.

Keeping scraping down the sides during the mixing procedure.

Heat a medium-sized pan over medium temperature.

When the pan is hot enough, pour in some of the melted butter.

Spread the butter evenly.

Use a ¼ cup measuring cup to ladle batter into the pan.

Swirl the batter around the pan to ensure it is equally distributed through the surface.

Cook the crepe until the bottom is firm and speckled with brown spots within 1 minute.

Now, loosen the edges and flip the crepe to cook the other side in the same time (1 minute).

Put on a plate when the crepe is speckled and golden on both sides.

Keep repeating this step until all the batter is used up.

When you are done, serve and enjoy.

Mediterranean grain bowl recipe with lentils and chickpeas

Ingredients

- 2 ½ tablespoons of fresh lemon juice
- Salt
- 1 zucchini squash, sliced into rounds
- 3 cups cooked faro
- 2 cups of cooked brown lentils
- 2 cups of cooked chickpeas
- ½ teaspoons of ground Sumac
- 2 ½ teaspoons of quality Dijon mustard
- 1 teaspoon of Za'atar spice
- Extra virgin olive oil
- 2 cups of cherry tomatoes, halved
- 2 shallots, sliced
- 1 cup of fresh chopped parsley
- Handful pitted Kalamata olives
- Sprinkle of crumbled feta cheese
- 2 avocados, skin removed, pitted and sliced
- 1 garlic clove, minced
- Salt and pepper

Directions

- In a skillet, heat 2 tablespoons of olive oil over medium heat until shimmering but without smoke.
- Add the sliced zucchini and sauté on both sides until tender.
- Remove zucchini and place on a paper towel to drain any excess oil.
- Season with salt.

- Add the extra virgin olive oil, lemon juice, garlic, salt and pepper, za'atar spice, and sumac to a mason jar.
- Close tightly, and give it a good shake. Set aside for later.
- Divide the cooked faro, lentils, and chickpeas equally among four dinner bowls.
- Add cooked zucchini, tomatoes, shallots, avocado slices, parsley, and Kalamata olives.
- Season with salt, pepper and za'atar then drizzle a bit of the dressing on top.
- Serve and enjoy at room temperature.

Roasted cauliflower and chickpea stew

This is a perfect match for serving over couscous or rice. The cauliflower is deliciously roasted and loaded with carrots, cumin, tomatoes, cinnamon and paprika for a Mediterranean dish.

Ingredients

- ½ cup of parsley leaves, stems removed, roughly chopped
- 1 ½ teaspoons of ground turmeric
- 1 28-oz. can of diced tomatoes with its juice
- 1 ½ teaspoons of ground cumin
- 1 ½ teaspoons of ground cinnamon
- 1 teaspoon of Sweet paprika
- Toasted pine nuts
- 2 14-oz. cans of chickpeas, drained and rinsed
- 1 teaspoon of cayenne pepper
- ½ teaspoon of ground green cardamom
- 1 whole head cauliflower, divided into small florets
- 5 medium-sized bulk carrots, peeled, cut pieces
- Salt and pepper
- Extra virgin olive oil
- Toasted slivered almonds
- 1 large sweet onion, chopped
- 1 teaspoon of ground coriander
- 6 garlic cloves, chopped

Directions

- Preheat the oven to 475°F.
- In a small bowl, mix together the spices.

- Place the cauliflower florets and carrot pieces on a large lightly oiled baking sheet.
- Season with salt and pepper.
- Add some spice mixture.
- Drizzle with olive oil, then toss to coat.
- Bake for 20 minutes in the preheated oven or until the carrots and cauliflower soften.
- Remove from the heat and keep for later. Turn the oven off.
- In a large cast iron pot , heat 2 tablespoons of olive oil.
- Add the onions and sauté for 3 minutes, add the garlic and the remaining spices.
- Let cook for 3 minutes on medium-high heat, stirring constantly.
- Add chickpeas with the canned tomatoes.
- Season with salt and pepper.
- Stir in the roasted cauliflower and carrots boil.
- Lower the heat, cover part-way let cook for 20 minutes.
- Transfer to serving bowls and garnish with fresh parsley.
- Serve and enjoy place over couscous.

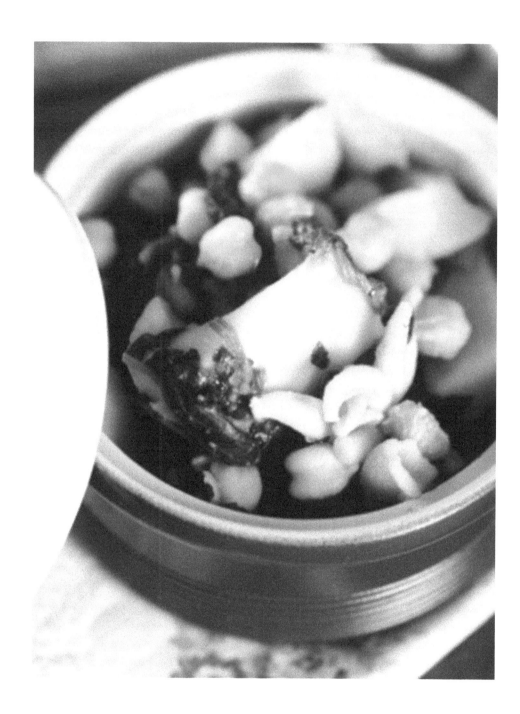

Jeweled couscous recipe with pomegranate and lentils

This recipe combines mushrooms, lentil, nuts and raisins for a gorgeous dish the Mediterranean Sea way for a vegan.

Ingredients

- Salt
- ½ teaspoon of turmeric spice
- Olive oil
- 8 oz. mushrooms, cleaned and sliced
- 3 garlic cloves, chopped
- 1 teaspoon of sweet paprika
- 1 ⅔ cup of vegetable broth
- Water
- ½ teaspoon of ground green cardamom
- ½ teaspoon of ground coriander
- 1 cup of lentils
- 1 cup of gold raisins
- ½ cup of shelled chopped pistachios
- ½ teaspoon of ground cumin
- 2 cups of instant couscous
- 1 bunch of fresh mint stems removed, chopped
- ½ teaspoon of freshly ground black pepper
- 2 tablespoons of pomegranate molasses
- Juice of ½ lemon
- 1 bunch of fresh parsley, stems removed, chopped
- 1 small red onion, chopped
- 1 ½ teaspoon of ground cinnamon
- 6 scallions, tops trimmed, chopped

- Seeds of 1 large pomegranate
- 10 Medjool dates , pitted, chopped

Directions

- Wash the lentils under running water. Drain.
- Place the lentils in a saucepan and add 3 cups of water let boil, then reduce to simmer for 30 minutes.
- Add a pinch of salt and remove from heat.
- In a saucepan, bring the vegetable broth to a boil.
- Stir in couscous together with the turmeric, pinch of salt, olive oil.
- Cover and let sit 5 minutes to finish cooking.
- In a large cast iron skillet, heat 2 tablespoons of olive oil.
- Add the mushrooms let cook for 4 minutes on high, tossing occasionally.
- Reduce heat to medium-high, and stir the onions and garlic and cook briefly.
- In the same skillet, add in the cooked lentils and couscous.
- Add salt together with the cinnamon, cardamom, paprika, coriander, and black pepper.
- Mix the pomegranate molasses and lemon juice with 1 tablespoon of olive oil.
- Add the liquid to the skillet with the couscous and lentil mixture. Toss to combine.
- Let cook on medium, stirring regularly to warm through.
- Remove from the heat, add the remaining ingredients.

- Move the couscous to a serving platter.
- Serve and enjoy.

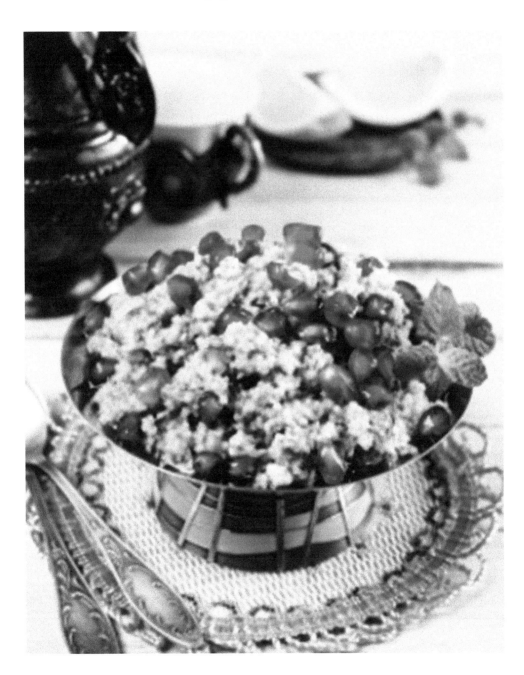

Easy Mediterranean style shrimp stew

This easy Mediterranean shrimp stew is prepared with chunky yet rustic tomato sauce with wonderful flavor from the garlic, onions, and bell peppers.

Ingredients

- ⅓ cup of toasted pine nuts, optional
- 1 large red onion, chopped
- 1 ½ teaspoon of ground coriander
- 1 bell pepper, cored, chopped
- 5 garlic cloves, chopped
- ¼ cup of toasted sesame seeds
- 1 teaspoon of sumac
- Extra virgin olive oil
- Lemon or lime wedges
- 1 teaspoon of red pepper flakes
- ½ teaspoon of ground green cardamom
- 2 15-oz. cans of diced tomatoes
- ½ cup water
- Kosher salt and black pepper
- 1 teaspoon of cumin
- 2 ½ lb. large shrimp
- 1 cup of parsley leaves

Directions

- Preheat the oven to 375°F.
- In a large skillet or frying pan, heat 2 tablespoons of extra virgin olive oil until shimmering but with smoke.
- Add chopped onions, bell peppers, and garlic.
- Let cook for 4 minutes, tossing regularly.
- Stir in spices and continue to cook for 1 more minute.

- Add diced tomatoes and water.
- Season with kosher salt and pepper.
- Boil, then lower heat to let simmer 15 minutes.
- Transfer sauce to an oven-save dish.
- Stir shrimp into the sauce.
- Add parsley together with the pine nuts, and toasted sesame seeds.
- Tighten the lid with a foil.
- Transfer to heated oven let bake for 9 minutes.
- Uncover and broil briefly till shrimp is ready.
- Serve and enjoy.

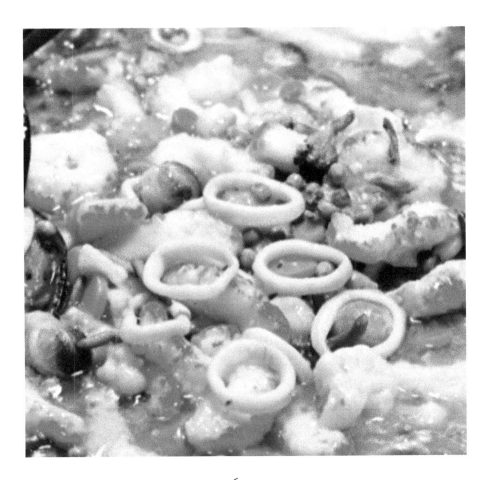

Extra creamy avocado hummus recipe

Avocado is the king for skin nourishing among Mediterranean Sea diet recipes. Chickpeas combined with creamy avocado will definitely surprise your taste buds every possible way flavored with garlic, cumin and cayenne.

Ingredients

- ½ lime, juice of lemon
- 2 garlic cloves
- 15-oz. can of chickpeas, drained
- Liquid from canned chickpeas
- ½ teaspoon of cayenne pepper
- 2 tablespoons of Greek Yogurt
- 3 tablespoons of tahini
- Salt
- 2 medium ripe avocados, roughly chopped
- 1 teaspoon of ground cumin

Directions

- In a large food processor, add the garlic together with the chickpeas, avocados, Greek yogurt, tahini, salt, cumin, cayenne and lime juice.
- Blend until the hummus mixture is smooth.
- Taste and adjust everything accordingly.
- Run the processor again until you achieve the desired creamy consistency. Again adjust seasoning as required.
- Transfer the avocado hummus to a serving dish and cover tightly with plastic wrap.
- Chill in a refrigerator before serving.

- Uncover and smooth the surface of the hummus and drizzle a bit of extra virgin olive oil.
- Garnish with fresh parsley.
- Serve and enjoy.

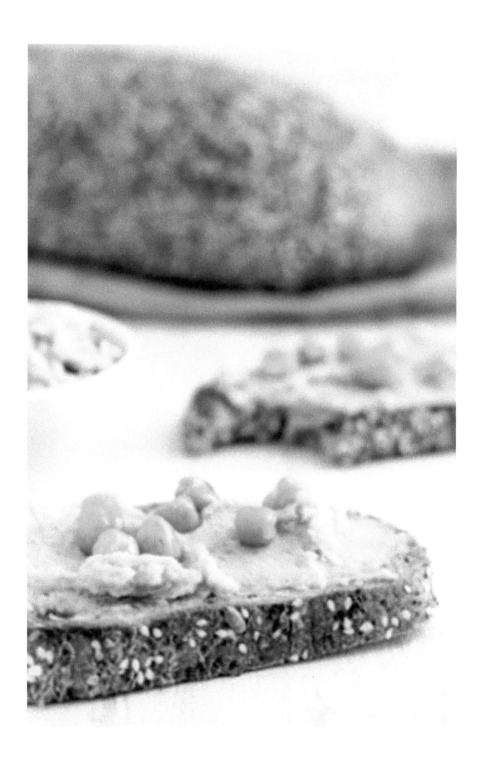

Melitzanosalata recipe

This recipe copes the Greek style of smoky dip of eggplant with aromatics especially garlic, parsley, lemon juice, and extra virgin olive oil.

Ingredients

- ¼ cup of extra virgin olive oil
- 2 large garlic cloves minced
- ¼ red onion finely chopped
- 2 large eggplants
- 1 cup of chopped fresh parsley packed
- Kosher salt and black pepper
- ½ teaspoon of each ground cumin
- A few pitted Kalamata olives sliced
- Feta cheese a sprinkle
- Crushed red pepper flakes
- 1 lemon zested and juiced

Directions

- Keep the eggplant whole and pierce with a fork in a few places.
- Place the eggplant over a gas flame or under a broiler, let cook, keep turning using tongs, until the skin is fully charred
- Cool and drain eggplant.
- Place the eggplant in a bowl and until cool enough to handle.
- Peel the charred skins off and discard.
- Cut into chunks and place in a colander to get rid of any remaining excess juices for 10 minutes.
- Shift eggplant to a mixing bowl.

- Add the garlic together with the onion, parsley, lemon juice, olive oil .
- Add salt and pepper and spices, mix to combine.
- Break up the eggplant into smaller chunks.
- Cover the eggplant dip well, let chill in the refrigerator shortly.
- Transfer the eggplant dip to a serving plate and spread.
- Drizzle with extra virgin olive oil.
- Organize and garnish with red onions, lemon zest, parsley, olives, a sprinkle of feta.
- Serve and enjoy with crusty bread.

Veggie teriyaki stir-fry with noodles

Quick and easy stir fry vegetables with noodles for a healthy dinner is perfect for a Mediterranean Sea diet in 40 minutes max.

Ingredients

- ½ cup teriyaki sauce
- ¼ cup thinly sliced green onion
- 2 tablespoons extra-virgin olive oil
- ½ teaspoon fine sea salt
- 6 cups thinly sliced mixed vegetables*
- 1 to 2 teaspoons toasted sesame oil
- 1 medium red or white onion
- 4 ounces soba noodles, brown rice noodles
- 1 teaspoon sesame seeds

Directions

- Bring a pot of water to boil.
- Place the noodles let cook the noodles as per the package Directions.
- Drain and set aside for later.
- Warm a large skillet over medium heat.
- Add the oil, onion, and salt let for 4 – 6 minutes until onions are tender.
- Add the remaining vegetables and cook until they are tender and caramelizing on the edges in 10 – 15 minutes.
- Add the noodles and ½ cup of teriyaki sauce to the pan.
- Stir to combine, let cook till the ingredients are all warmed through in 1 minute.
- Remove the skillet from the heat source.

- Add toasted sesame oil together with the sesame seeds.
- Serve the noodles in bowls with sliced green onion.
- Sprinkle with sesame seeds on top.
- Serve and enjoy.

Roasted butternut squash, pomegranate and wild rice stuffing

The recipe can take up to 1 hour and 20 minutes but the sweetness and the health benefit achieved from eating it makes it worth waiting for. It is prepared with kale, wild rice and pomegranate serving from 6 – 12 servings.

Ingredients
- Arils from 1 medium pomegranate,
- 1 tablespoon of maple syrup
- 1 tablespoon of Dijon mustard
- 4 ounces of kale, ribs removed and chopped
- ¾ cup of chopped green onion
- 1 tablespoon of grated fresh ginger
- ½ cup of raw pepitas
- 1 teaspoon of extra-virgin olive oil
- 2 teaspoon of fine sea salt
- 2 tablespoons of apple cider vinegar
- 2 cups of wild rice
- ¼ teaspoon ground cinnamon
- 1 small-to-medium butternut squash
- 2 teaspoon of fine sea salt
- 4 ounces of goat cheese
- ¼ cup of extra-virgin olive oil

Directions
- Preheat your oven to 425°F.
- Line a large baking sheet with parchment paper.
- Bring a large pot of water to boil.
- Add the rice let cook under reducing heat to simmer for 40 – 55 minutes.

- Remove from heat, drain, return the rice to the pot
- Place the cubed butternut squash onto the baking sheet.
- Drizzle it with the olive oil and a sprinkle of salt.
- Toss until the cubes are lightly and evenly coated in oil.
- Arrange them in single layer let roast for 35 – 50 minutes tossing occasionally.
- Chop the kale and green onion, remove the arils from the pomegranate, whisk together dressing ingredients in a small bowl.
- combine the pepitas with 1 teaspoon olive oil, ¼ teaspoon of salt and cinnamon in a small skillet stir. Cook for 3 – 5 minutes.
- Stir in half of the green onions, kale, and ginger dressing.
- Spread the mixture over a large serving platter.
- Arrange the butternut squash over the wild rice mixture.
- Crumble the goat cheese on top with a fork.
- Top with the toasted pepitas, pomegranate arils, and green onions.
- Serve while warm and enjoy.

Crispy bean tostadas with smashed avocado and jicama-cilantro slaw

The beans are refried the Mexican way with avocado and cabbage slaw crisp. Prepared with fillings entirely meatless perfect for a Mediterranean Sea diet.

Ingredients

- ½ medium red onion, thinly sliced
- Salt
- Juice of 2 lime
- 6 corn of tortillas
- 2 cups shredded green cabbage
- ½ cup of crumbled queso fresco
- ½ teaspoon ground cumin
- Freshly ground black pepper
- ½ cup fresh cilantro leaves
- Extra-virgin olive oil
- 2 cans of vegetarian refried beans
- 1 tablespoon white vinegar
- ½ teaspoon chili powder
- 3 large ripe avocados, pitted and peeled
- ½ cup ¼-inch-thick slices peeled jicama
- ½ cup of halved grape tomatoes

Directions

- In a medium bowl, combine the sliced onions together with the lime juice, vinegar and salt stir to coated the onions set aside.
- In a large bowl, combine the cilantro, cabbage, lime juice, jicama, cumin and chili powder.
- Season with salt and pepper accordingly.
- Preheat your oven to 425°F.

- Brush both sides of the tortilla with olive oil let season with salt.
- Organize in a single layer on a large baking sheet.
- Bake for 4 minutes, flip and bake for 4 – 8 minutes, till crispy.
- Gently heat the refried beans in the microwave.
- In a large sized bowl, mash the avocados with a fork.
- Stir in the lime juice and season with salt accordingly.
- Spread refried beans evenly over every tortilla.
- Add a layer of smashed avocado and top with the pickled onions, slaw, tomatoes and queso fresco.
- Serve soon enough and enjoy.

Mango burrito bowls with crispy tofu and peanut sauce

The recipe is prepared with tofu, brown rice, peanut sauce and fresh mango from the tree. It takes max I hour and 15 minutes to get ready.

Ingredients
- ½ cup of sliced green onions
- 1 block of organic extra-firm tofu
- 1 medium red bell pepper, chopped
- 1 tablespoon extra-virgin olive oil
- ¼ cup chopped fresh cilantro
- 3 tablespoon reduced-sodium tamari
- 2 cups shredded cabbage
- ¼ teaspoon fine sea salt
- 1 tablespoon cornstarch
- 1 medium jalapeño, seeds and ribs removed, minced
- 1 ¼ cups brown basmati rice
- ⅓ cup creamy peanut butter
- 5 tablespoons lime juice
- 1 tablespoon honey or maple syrup, to taste
- 2 teaspoons toasted sesame oil
- Handful of chopped roasted peanuts
- 2 garlic cloves, minced
- ¼ teaspoon red pepper flakes
- 2 large ripe mangos

Directions
- Preheat your oven to 400°F.
- Align a large baking sheet with parchment paper.

- Drain the tofu.
- Slice the tofu into thirds lengthwise in 3 even slabs.
- Stack the slabs on top of each other and slice through them lengthwise to 3 even columns, slice across to 5 even rows.
- Arrange the tofu in an even layer on a board with towels.
- Fold the towel over the cubed tofu.
- Place something heavy on top to drain.
- Allow it to rest for at least 10 minutes or accordingly.
- Bring a large pot of water to boil.
- Add the rice, boil uncovered for 30 minutes.
- Drain and return the rice to the pot.
- Cover the pot let rice simmer for 10 minutes, set aside.
- Move the pressed tofu to the lined baking sheet.
- Drizzle with the olive oil and tamari.
- Toss to combine and sprinkle the starch over the tofu toss again till evenly coated.
- Arrange the tofu in an even layer.
- Bake for 25 – 30 minutes toss halfway, until deeply golden on the edges. Set aside.
- Whisk all the ingredients together in a bowl.
- Taste and season accordingly, set aside.
- In a medium mixing bowl, combine the diced mango, bell pepper, green jalapeño, onion, lime juice, cilantro, and salt.
- Stir to combine, and set aside.

- Scoop rice top with a handful of shredded cabbage.
- Add a big scoop of mango salsa, a handful of baked tofu, a hefty drizzle of peanut sauce, and a sprinkle of chopped peanuts.
- Serve and enjoy

Halloumi tacos with pineapple salsa and aji Verde

Ingredients

- Aji Verde
- 8 small corn
- ¼ cup of extra-virgin olive oil
- Pineapple Salsa
- 8 ounces of halloumi cheese, sliced into rounds

Directions

- In a medium skillet using a medium heat, warm the tortilla through.
- Stack them together under a clean tea towel.
- In the same skillet, warm olive oil over medium heat.
- Place slices of halloumi into the hot oil.
- Cook the cheese until golden in 2 – 4 minutes.
- Flip each piece of cheese with the tongs let cook until the other side is golden 2 – 4 minutes.
- Place a few paper towels on a cutting board to absorb excess oil.
- Place cooked cheese onto the plate let cool a bit before handling.
- Slice each piece of cheese into strips.
- Place a few strips of cheese along half of your tortilla.
- Top with pineapple salsa.
- Finish each taco with a drizzle of aji Verde.
- Serve warm and enjoy.

Baked ziti with roasted vegetables

Roasted vegetables are significant in elevating this baked ziti. Prepared with mozzarella, pasta and red sauce, the baked ziti with roasted vegetables is a delicious meal.

Ingredients

- 2 cups of cottage cheese
- 1 red bell pepper
- 8 ounces of ziti, rigatoni
- 2 tablespoons of extra-virgin olive oil
- ¼ teaspoon of fine sea salt
- 1 medium head of cauliflower cut into florets
- 4 cups of marinara sauce
- ¼ cup of chopped fresh basil
- 1 medium yellow onion, wedged
- 8 ounces of grated part-skim mozzarella cheese

Directions

- Preheat your oven to 425°F.
- Line two large baking sheets with parchment paper.
- Place the cauliflower florets on one pan.
- Combine the bell peppers and onion on the other.
- Drizzle olive oil over the pans.
- Sprinkle salt over the two pans.
- Toss until the vegetables on each pan are lightly coated in oil.
- Organize the vegetables in an even layer across each pan.
- Bake for 30 – 35 minutes till the vegetables are tender and caramelized on the edges.

- Toss the veggies and swapping their rack positions halfway.
- Bring a large pot of salted water to boil.
- Cook the pasta according to package instruction.
- Drain and return to the pot.
- Add 2 cups of the marinara, the chopped basil, and ½ cup of the mozzarella, stir to combine.
- Spread 1 cup of marinara sauce inside the baker.
- Top with half of the pasta mixture, spread into an even layer.
- Sprinkle the roasted cauliflower on top.
- Dollop 1 cup of the cottage cheese over the cauliflower and ½ cup of the mozzarella.
- Top with the remaining pasta.
- Sprinkle the roasted peppers and onion on top.
- Dollop the remaining cup of ricotta and marina.
- Sprinkle the remaining cheese all over.
- Place the baking sheet on the lower oven rack to catch any drippings.
- Place the ziti, uncovered, on top of the baking sheet.
- Bake for 30 minutes
- Move to the upper rack for 2 – 5 minutes until deeply golden
- Remove the baker from the oven let cool for 10 minutes.
- Sprinkle freshly torn basil on top, slice with a knife.
- Serve and enjoy.

Thai panang curry vegetables

The recipe embraces the health power of vegetable; as such, it is fully packed with vegetables and variety of fresh flavors.

Ingredients
- Fresh Thai basil, sriracha or chili garlic sauce
- 1 tablespoon coconut oil
- 1 to 2 tablespoons panang curry paste
- 1 tablespoon tamari
- Pinch of salt
- ½ cup water
- 1 yellow, orange, sliced into strips
- 3 carrots, peeled and sliced
- 2 cloves garlic, pressed
- 1 can regular coconut milk
- 2 tablespoons peanut butter
- 1 ½ teaspoons coconut sugar
- 1 red bell pepper, sliced into strips
- 1 small white or yellow onion, chopped
- 2 teaspoons fresh lime juice

Directions
- Bring a large pot of water to boil.
- Add rice boil for 30 minutes, lower heat and simmer.
- When ready drain, return the rice to pot.
- Cover let rest for 10 minutes set aside.
- Warm a large skillet over medium heat.
- When hot, add the oil with onion and a sprinkle of salt let cook, stirring often for 5 minutes.

- Add bell peppers and carrots let cook until bell peppers can be pierced with fork 3 – 5 minutes, stirring occasionally.
- Add the garlic and curry paste
- Let cook for 1 minute, while stirring.
- Add coconut milk together with water, stir to combine.
- Simmer the mixture over medium heat.
- Adjust the heat as necessary until the peppers and carrots have softened in 5 – 10 minutes, stirring occasionally.
- Remove the pot from the heat.
- Stir in the peanut butter, sugar, tamari, and lime juice.
- Add salt and season accordingly.
- Divide rice and curry into bowls and garnish with fresh basil.
- Serve and enjoy.

Crispy baked tofu

Ingredients
- 1 block of organic extra-firm tofu
- 1 tablespoon of extra-virgin olive oil
- 1 tablespoon of tamari
- 1 tablespoon of cornstarch

Directions
- Start by preheat your oven to 400°F.
- Align a large baking sheet with parchment paper.
- Drain the tofu with you palms to gently squeeze out the water.
- Slice the tofu into thirds lengthwise.
- Stack the slabs on top of each other and slice through them lengthwise making 3 even columns.
- Slice across to make 5 even rows.
- Get a chopping board with towel.
- Arrange the tofu in an even layer on the towel cover with a heavy object to drain extra water.
- Move pressed tofu to a medium mixing bowl
- Drizzle with the olive oil and tamari.
- Toss to combine.
- Sprinkle the starch over the tofu, toss until starch is evenly coated.
- Bake for 25 – 30 minutes, toss halfway, until deeply golden on edges.
- Serve and enjoy.

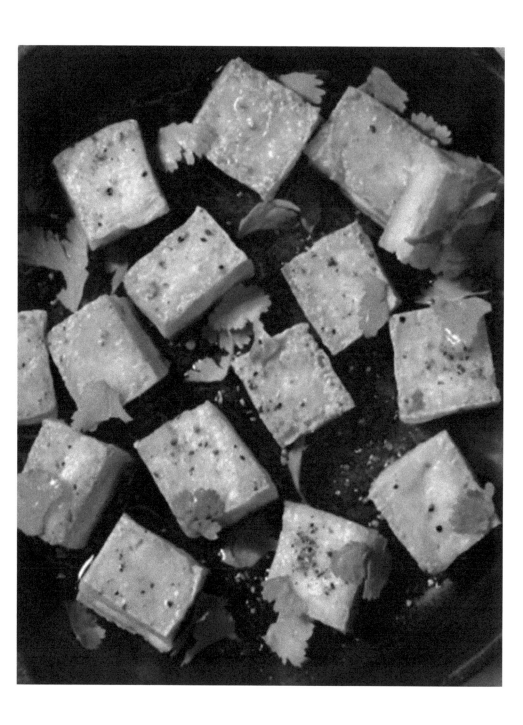

Homemade veggie chili

This recipe features smoky and complex flavors. It emerged from poultry ingredients and vegetable varieties and classic spices to spike its sweetness and delicacy.

Ingredients

- 2 ribs celery, chopped
- ½ teaspoon salt
- 4 cloves garlic, pressed
- Tortilla chips
- 2 tablespoons chili powder
- 1 ½ teaspoons smoked paprika
- 1 teaspoon dried oregano
- 2 tablespoons extra-virgin olive oil
- Sour cream
- 1 large can of diced tomatoes
- 2 cans of black beans, rinsed and drained
- 1 medium red onion, chopped
- 1 large red bell pepper, chopped
- 1 can of pinto beans, rinsed and drained
- Sliced avocado
- 2 cups of vegetable broth
- 1 bay leaf
- 2 medium carrots, chopped
- 2 tablespoons chopped fresh cilantro
- 1 to 2 teaspoons sherry vinegar
- 2 teaspoons ground cumin
- Chopped cilantro

Directions

- In a large oven warm the olive oil until shimmering without smoke over medium heat.
- Add the chopped bell pepper, onion, celery, carrot, and ¼ teaspoon of the salt stir to combine.
- Cook until the vegetables are tender, onion translucent in 7 – 10 minutes, stirring occasionally.
- Add garlic, cumin, chili powder, smoked paprika and oregano.
- Cook until fragrant, stirring constantly for 1 minute.
- Add diced tomatoes, black beans, vegetable broth, pinto beans, and bay leaf.
- Stir to combine then simmer for 30 minutes.
- Remove the chili from the heat and discard the bay leaf.
- Move 1 ½ cups of the chili to a blender, blend till smooth.
- Pour the mixture back into the pot.
- Add the chopped cilantro, stir to combine.
- Stir in the vinegar to taste.
- Add salt accordingly.
- Place in bowls serve and enjoy.

Vegetarian stuffed acorn squash

The use of quinoa filling gives this recipe a beautifully tasty flavor that you cannot possibly resist.

Ingredients
- ¼ cup raw pepitas
- ¼ cup chopped green onion
- 1 cup water
- 2 tablespoons extra-virgin olive oil
- ¼ cup chopped parsley
- 1 clove garlic minced
- 2 medium acorn squash
- ½ teaspoon fine sea salt
- 1 tablespoon lemon juice
- ¾ cup grated Parmesan cheese
- ½ cup quinoa, rinsed
- ¼ cup dried cranberries
- ½ cup crumbled goat cheese

Directions
- Preheat the oven to 400°F.
- Align a large baking sheet with parchment paper.
- Slice through the squash up to down, scoop out the seeds and stringy bits inside.
- Place the squash halves on the parchment pan.
- Drizzle 1 tablespoon of the olive oil over the squash.
- Sprinkle with ¼ teaspoon of salt.

- Rub the oil into the cut sides of the squash, face the cut sides to the pan.
- Bake until squash is easily pierced through in 30 – 45 minutes.
- In a separate medium saucepan, combine quinoa with water.
- Boil over medium-high heat, then lower heat to simmer uncovered for 12 – 18 minutes.
- Stir in the cranberries when the mixture is off heat.
- Cover let steam for 5 minutes.
- In a medium skillet, toast the pepitas over medium heat as you keep stirring frequently, until golden on the edges in 4 – 5 minutes. Keep aside.
- Put the quinoa mixture into a medium mixing bowl.
- Add the toasted garlic, pepitas, parsley, onion, lemon juice, the remaining ¼ teaspoon of salt, and 1 tablespoon of olive oil.
- Stir for even distribution.
- Taste and season accordingly.
- Add the Parmesan cheese and goat cheese stir to combine.
- Turn the cooked squash halves over.
- Divide the mixture evenly between halves a spoon.
- Return the squash to the oven let bake for 15 – 18 minutes.

- Sprinkle the stuffed squash with 1 tablespoon of chopped parsley.
- Serve warm and enjoy.

Crispy falafel

Ingredients

- ½ teaspoon of ground cumin
- ¼ cup and 1 tablespoon extra-virgin olive oil
- 1 teaspoon of fine sea salt
- ¼ teaspoon of ground cinnamon
- ½ cup of roughly chopped red onion
- ½ cup of packed fresh cilantro
- ½ teaspoon of freshly ground black pepper
- ½ cup of packed fresh parsley
- 1 cup of dried chickpeas

Directions

- Preheat oven to 375 °F.
- Pour ¼ cup of the olive oil in a large baking sheet tilt round to evenly coat.
- Combine chickpeas, onion, garlic, parsley, salt, pepper, cilantro, cumin, cinnamon, and 1 tablespoon of olive oil in a food processor. Blend for 1 minute till smooth.
- Shape the falafel into small patties, 2 inches wide, ½ inch thick.
- Place them falafel on the oiled pan.
- Bake for 25 – 30 minutes ensure to flip over to bake all sides.
- Serve and enjoy.

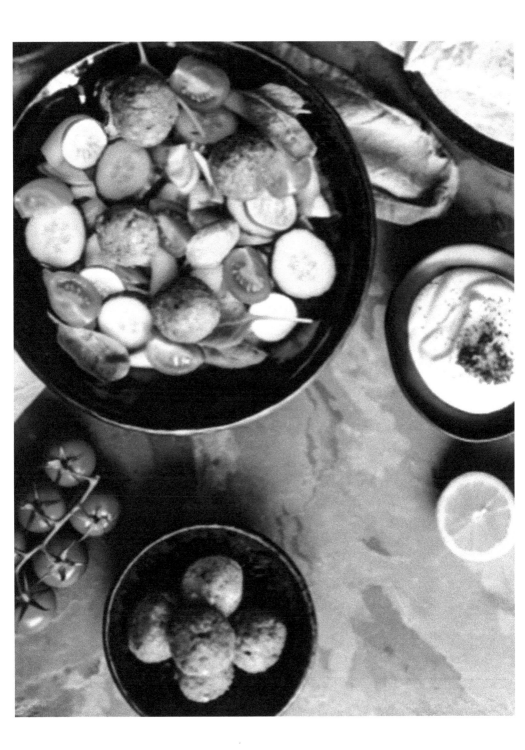

Epic vegetarian tacos

Using pickled onions, refried beans, and avocado sauce, this recipe is so delightfully delicious for a meal with meatless tacos.

Ingredients

- Creamy avocado dip
- 8 corn tortillas
- Quick-pickled onions
- Chopped fresh cilantro
- Lime wedges
- Salsa Verde
- Shredded green cabbage
- Crumbled Cotjia
- Easy refried beans

Directions

- Prepare these ingredients normally onions, avocado dip, and beans.
- In a large skillet, warm every side of the tortillas over medium temperature in batches.
- Stack the warmed tortillas on a plate and cover.
- Spread refried beans down but at the center of every tortilla.
- Top with avocado dip and onions.
- Garnish and serve.
- Enjoy.

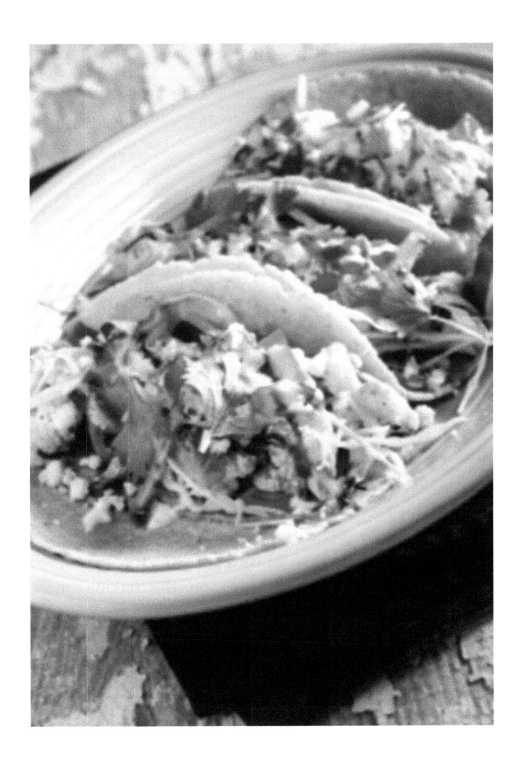

Loaded vegetables nachos

This is a quicker Mediterranean Sea diet veggies with zero percent meat. Prepared with creamy avocado sauce and cheese in 25 minutes.

Ingredients
- 1 packed cup of shredded cheddar cheese
- red bell pepper, chopped
- ⅓ cup crumbled feta cheese
- Your favorite salsa
- 1 can of pinto beans, rinsed and drained
- Avocado dip
- ⅓ cup chopped green onions
- 1 packed cup of shredded Monterey Jack cheese
- 2 radishes, chopped
- Pickled jalapeños
- 2 tablespoons chopped cilantro

Directions
- Begin by preheating your oven to 400°F.
- Align a baking sheet with parchment paper.
- Place handfuls of chips on the baking sheet distributed evenly.
- Sprinkle the prepared pan of chips evenly with the beans and so the shredded cheese, crumbled feta, bell pepper, and pickled jalapeños.
- Bake until the cheese is melted in 9 − 13 minutes.
- When ready, remove, set aside.

- Drizzle the nachos with avocado sauce.
- Sprinkle the nachos with radish, onion, and cilantro.
- Serve soon enough and enjoy when still warm.

Pinto posole

The vegetarian type pinto posole features beans instead of pork.

This recipe is spicy, flavorful and delicious to light up your taste buds.

Ingredients

- ½ teaspoon fine sea salt
- 2 tablespoons extra-virgin olive oil
- 1 lime, halved
- 1 tablespoon ground cumin
- ½ cup of tomato paste
- 1 bay leaf
- 2 cups water
- 3 cans of pinto beans, rinsed and drained
- 2 to 4 guajillo chili peppers
- 1 can of hominy, rinsed and drained
- 32 ounces of vegetable broth
- 4 cloves garlic, pressed or minced
- 1 large white onion, finely chopped
- ¼ cup chopped cilantro

Directions

- Heat your oven over a medium heat until it evaporates.
- Toast the chili press flat with a spatula briefly till fragrant flip over repeat.
- In the same pot, warm the olive oil until shimmering without smoke.

- Add the onion and a pinch of salt.
- Cook while stirring frequently, until onions turn translucent in 5 minutes.
- Add the garlic together with cumin let cook until fragrant in 1 minute.
- Add the tomato paste cook for 1 minute, keep stirring.
- Add toasted chili peppers, hominy, bay leaf, vegetable broth, beans, and water to the pot.
- Stir in salt and raise the heat to medium.
- Simmer regulate the heat for 25 minutes.
- Discard the chili peppers and bay leaf..
- Stir the cilantro and juice of lime into the soup.
- Taste and season accordingly.
- Garnish with lime wedges.
- Serve and enjoy.

Real stovetop mac and cheese

Ingredients

- Tiny pinch of cayenne pepper
- ⅓ cup of heavy cream
- 1 ⅓ packed cups of sharp cheddar cheese
- 8 ounces of regular macaroni noodles
- ⅛ teaspoon of onion powder
- ½ teaspoon of mustard powder
- 2 teaspoons of salt
- ⅛ teaspoon of garlic powder

Directions

- Bring water to boil in a medium pot.
- Add noodles and salt.
- Let cook according to package Directions.
- Drain the pasta let stay in the colander.
- Return the same pot heat.
- Add cream let boil time for 1 minute.
- Add cheese with spices when the timer is up, stir till cheese has melted.
- Add boiled pasta, stir to coated in cheese sauce.
- Remove the pot from the heat source.
- Taste and season accordingly.
- Best served and enjoyed immediately.

Super simple marinara sauce

With only 5 core ingredients, this marinara sauce is quite simple to make yet very delicious. Here, there is no struggle in chopping this and that because it is not needed.

Ingredients
- Salt
- 1 medium yellow onion
- 2 large cloves garlic left whole
- Pinch of red pepper flakes
- 1 large can of whole peeled tomatoes
- 1 teaspoon of dried oregano
- 2 tablespoons of extra-virgin olive oil

Directions
- Combine tomatoes, garlic cloves, olive oil, halved onion, oregano and red pepper flakes in a medium saucepan.
- Simmer over low heat for 45 minutes.
- Stir occasionally, crush tomatoes with the back of a spoon.
- Take off the pot from heat source, throw the onion.
- Stir smashed garlic into the sauce.
- Add salt season to taste.
- Serve warm and enjoy.
- Leftover can be refrigerated for later consumption.

Hearty spaghetti with lentils and marinara

This is a recipe for typical whole meal with lentils, spaghetti, variety of vegetables, and marinara sauce for lunch or dinner. It comes delightfully delicious in only 35 minutes. You can surely wait for that times. Don't you?

Ingredients

- 8 ounces of whole-grain pasta
- 1 bay leaf

- 2 cups of marinara sauce
- 1 large garlic clove, left whole
- ¼ teaspoon of salt
- ½ cup of dry lentils
- 2 cups of vegetable broth

Directions

- In a small saucepan, combine the bay leaf, garlic, lentils, salt, and broth.
- Simmer over medium-high heat for 20 – 35 minutes till the lentils have cooked through.
- Drain the lentils, throw away bay leaf and garlic. Keep uncovered.
- Boil salted water in a large saucepan.
- Place in the pasta, cook according to package instruction.
- Drain, return to the pot keep.

- Stir the marinara into the lentils, warm over medium heat.
- Divide pasta into bowls.
- Top with warm marinara and lentils.
- Serve and enjoy warm.

Creamy pumpkin marinara

In a period of 25 minutes, this recipe will be read. It readily tastes like fall with comfort just like mac with cheese stuffed with variety of vegetables; of course it is a Mediterranean Sea diet, do not expect anything less vegetarian,

Ingredients

- Finely grated Parmesan and chopped parsley
- 1 red bell pepper, chopped
- ½ teaspoon of dried oregano
- 2 teaspoons of balsamic vinegar
- ¼ teaspoon of dried tarragon
- ¼ teaspoon of ground cinnamon
- 1 can of diced tomatoes
- 1 can of pumpkin purée
- ½ teaspoon of salt, divided
- 2 tablespoons of butter
- 2 cloves garlic, minced
- 2 tablespoons of extra-virgin olive oil
- 1 yellow onion, chopped
- Freshly ground black pepper

Directions

- In a large skillet, warm olive oil over medium heat.
- Let shimmer without smoke.
- Add onion, bell pepper and salt.
- Let cook while stirring frequently, till onions and pepper are tender in 8 minutes.

- Add garlic, tarragon, oregano, and cinnamon let cook for 1 minute.
- Introduce tomatoes let cook for 1 minute.
- Stir in the pumpkin purée, stir to combine.
- Simmering for 5 minutes over low heat.
- Move the mixture to a blender.
- Add 1 butter together with the vinegar.
- Blend until very smooth.
- Season with ground black pepper and salt.
- Stir in the warm pasta.
- Serve with grated Parmesan and chopped parsley.
- Enjoy

Steel cut oat risotto with butternut squash and kale

Ingredients

- 1 ½ cups of Quaker steel-cut oats
- 1 teaspoon salt
- 2 packed cups chopped kale
- ½ cup dry white wine
- Freshly ground black pepper
- 6 cups water
- 1 small butternut squash
- 1 medium red onion, chopped
- ¾ cup of freshly grated Parmesan cheese
- 2 tablespoons butter
- 2 tablespoons extra-virgin olive oil
- 1 tablespoon lemon juice
- Pinch of red pepper flakes
- 4 cloves garlic or minced

Directions

- Warm olive oil until shimmering without smoke in a medium sized oven.
- Add butternut, onion, salt, and red pepper flakes.
- Let cook until the onion is translucent in 8 – 10 minutes.
- Add garlic together with oats, kale cook to combine in 2 minutes while stirring.

- Add the wine and scape up with silicone spatula till brown bits form at the bottom.
- Continue to cook for more 2 minutes keep stirring.
- Add water and remaining salt.
- Increased the heat to high let it boil.
- Lower the heat to allow simmering for 20 – 30 minutes. Ensure the bottom does not scorch
- Stir in the butter, Parmesan, lemon juice and black pepper.
- Let rest for 5 minutes.
- Divide in bowls, serve and enjoy.

Lightning Source UK Ltd.
Milton Keynes UK
UKHW020758030621
384857UK00005B/61